Blushing Breakthrough: How to Stop Blushing and Conquer Social Anxiety

Second Edition

© 2009 Jim Baker

ISBN #: 978-0-557-29688-0

FOREWORD

CONGRATULATIONS! You've just taken your first step to overcoming your blushing problem!

You may think that I'm talking about buying this book, and to an extent, I am, but that's not the first step to becoming a more social- **and less socially anxious-** person. While this book is a great way to help you face your fears and tackle your issues head on, this is just a helpful tool to help you find your path. No, you've taken the first step without this book, without me, and without anyone else helping you. Millions of people around the globe have trouble making the commitment to this crucial first step, and hold themselves back from making the full recovery that they deserve!

So what exactly is this first step? You probably aren't even aware that you've taken it. You're probably thinking that you have a long way to go before you notice any progress with your problem, but **you're wrong!**

You see, by taking the initiative and buying this book, you are indicating two things:

1. **You recognize you have an issue!**

    Everybody in today's world seems totally focused on themselves: me, me, me! With this type of global atmosphere, it can be really easy to fall into the trap and blame your social anxiety on the rest of the world instead of yourself. This may seem obvious to you, but you would be surprised at how many people with the same problem try to blame society, or the world, or even God for their problems. By buying this book, you inherently recognize that **you are the problem and have no one else to blame:** not your parents, not society, and not the world.

2. **You recognize that you think there is a solution!**

    This is absolutely integral to recovery. One of the worst things you can do to yourself is think that you were born defectively or that something is permanently wrong with you. This is just how our bodies work. If we have depression or anxiety, then our brains tend to tell us to feel sorry for ourselves. Somebody who feels like this may think that this is just the way that nature works, and they are stuck feeling anxious and blushing every time a social situation arises.

But this just isn't true! We are humanity, the greatest race on the planet, and we can conquer our nature. We tend to feel sorry for ourselves for simple biological reasons, and simple biological reasons cannot stop us!

Recognizing that your problem isn't a chronic condition that you will have to deal with for the rest of your life is an enormous leap of faith and confidence-- qualities that you will absolutely need if you want to have a full recovery! People who think that there is no hope for a cure tend to make self-fulfilling prophecies. They think that they cannot recover and begin leading a normal life, so they cannot. The sad truth is that, for most people, this negative thought is one of the only things stopping them from recovering. It's a cruel cycle – believe me, I know- but it's one that can easily be broken.

You bought this book because you thought that there was a solution to your problem. If you didn't think, on some level, that your condition was curable, then you wouldn't have wasted your money and would have simply kept going on feeling sorry for yourself. But you bought this book, thinking that maybe somebody, somewhere, had the tools to improve your life and help you overcome your blushing problem. This type of positive, proactive attitude is priceless, and is a major first step in the recovery process.

So, again, **congratulations!** You've already come a lot further than many of your fellow blushers, and a new life is in sight! Does this mean that you can put the book down and go out into the world right now? Probably not. Depending on how severe your condition is, overcoming blushing and social anxiety can take a lot of work. But a positive attitude is absolutely critical to approaching these tasks, especially when the going gets tough.

Fortunately, this book has all the tools you need to get you on your feet and get you moving. From explaining the reasons for blushing and social anxiety to giving you easy tips and tricks for helping you become the person you always wanted to be, this book has the answers that you seek.

Becoming a socially healthy person is easier than you think, and it's something that you, as a human being, deserve. Keep reading and good luck on your journey!

CHAPTER ONE

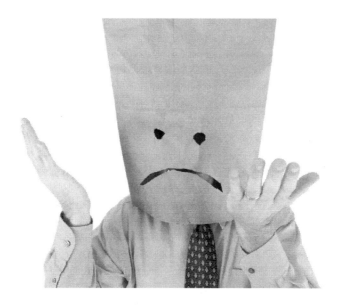

INTRODUCTION

A Blusher's Story

So, who exactly am I to tell you how to overcome the blushing demon and begin living a normal life? After all, I'm not a scientist or a leading psychologist. Why do I have the secret to the tools you will need to recover? The answer is simple: motivation. Researchers and therapists don't have the level of motivation to find a cure to blushing because they didn't suffer from it on such an intense and daily basis like I did. Allow me to tell you a story that may sound very familiar:

It was the day of a big date. Hours before, I told myself over and over that I would not blush. After all, my blushing had ruined countless dates before, and this was a particularly cute and friendly woman who I really wanted to impress. I spent a few hours in front of the mirror, trying to concentrate on not blushing, praying that I wouldn't blush. Any day but today, I thought. If I don't blush, then she will see me for who I really am and there won't be a problem at all. If only I wouldn't blush!

Needless to say, this line of thinking got me very nervous. My palms began to sweat, and my heart was racing uncontrollably. I took a hot shower and tried to relax myself, but all I could think about is that I would inevitably start blushing.

I waited in front of the restaurant, like we had agreed, and was so uncontrollably nervous that I began to blush before she had even arrived. Imagine how I felt, a huge blushing mess just standing there turning red all by himself. When she finally did arrive (and it felt like forever!) she came up to me and kissed me on the cheek. She was very friendly and inviting, and didn't give me any reason to feel nervous, but there I was, blushing like a fool.

"How are you?" she said. It was raining outside and she didn't quite have a good look at my face, but I started panicking. *Oh god*, I thought. *She sees that my face is a big tomato.*

"Uhh, I, Uhhh, umm, hi, hello" is what dribbled out of my incoherently stumbling lips. She flashed a friendly smile, but I knew that she knew that I was a nervous wreck.

"Shall we go in?" she asked. I wasn't thinking about the restaurant, though. My tunnel-vision mind was fixated on the fact that she knew she was going on a date with a blusher. *She knows*, I kept thinking over and over. *She knows!*

I don't quite remember how I got into the restaurant at that point, but somehow I did, and found myself at the table, sitting across from her. She was a nice woman, and very pretty, and a thought entered my mind that I could very well be having a very nice time right now. But I felt my cheeks burning as usual, and knew that I was a terrible blushing wreck. The restaurant's lighting had no chance of concealing my malaise.

She was starting to get uncomfortable as well. She had began the night smiling, but after seeing that all I could do was sit and blush, she started looking around the room anxiously. When the waiter came to take our order, I had a very difficult time focusing on the menu. She ordered something, maybe it was the salmon (I don't remember well), and I was staring down at the menu to see what I wanted but I simply could not concentrate. I was reading the words on the menu, but they didn't have any meaning.

I ended up nervously chirping "Me too!" when the waiter came for my order.

"Me too, sir?" The waiter said. *Oh god oh god, he knows I'm blushing too!*

"Y-yes!" I said.

The waiter gave me a funny look. I can tell you that this did not help my situation.

"So, you're having whatever the lady is having? Is that what you mean?" he said coldly. He hates me, I know it.

I simply shook my head in agreement. He walked off, smirking.

I was simply so overwhelmed with nervous energy that I couldn't sit still. Nervously, I excused myself and went to the men's room. Of course, this was a terrible mistake, because men's rooms have mirrors, which gave me a great view of my blood-red colored face. The restaurant was kept very cool, yet the room felt sweltering hot. It felt like every blood vessel that I had rushed straight up and had attached themselves to my cheeks. I tried to relax myself, and I splashed water on my face and tried to breathe deeply. It took me a few minutes, but I finally thought that I had the situation under control. I walked out of the bathroom and back to the table.

Only she was gone. She had walked out of the restaurant and left me with the empty table. I could see the waiter out of the corner of my eye. He knew what had happened. He was judging me. I felt every blood vessel in my face bulge. I was as bright-red as ever. Not knowing what else to do, I stormed out of the restaurant and ran all the way back to my home.

I had an issue with blushing before this incident, but this date just pushed me right over the edge. I began to feel very negative about my condition and myself. I felt that something was uncontrollably wrong with me, that I was somehow a defective human, and I began to feel very sorry for myself. I started withdrawing from friends and family, and began calling out of work more and more often. My employer began to get worried, and called my family to express his concern. Even though all these people cared for me and looked out for me, I didn't want to hear any of it. All I could focus on was my intense hatred of blushing.

I knew that I had to cure myself of this malady. I longed desperately to be a socially accepted person, to be well-liked and to feel like a member of the pack. I was unwilling to continue my life as a hermit. I had to do something. I felt like I could easily participate in society and become a likable, popular human being. If only my face didn't light up like a Christmas decoration every time I encountered another person!

At this time, I was willing to try everything, and so I did. At first, I tried to wear makeup to cover my face. I went out and had a custom skin toner made for my pigmentation. I put on a thick coat of this and tried to walk out into the public. I looked like a complete clown, but I didn't particularly care, as long as it didn't look like I was blushing. I quickly realized, however, that this simply made me look like an idiot wearing makeup and who was unable to control his blushing. I literally looked like a rosy-cheeked circus clown. I also realized that, even if it covered my blushing, wearing such a thick layer of makeup made me seem just as strange (if not stranger) than someone with a blushing problem. So I threw out my makeup, and all of the money I had spent on it went along as well.

 I started getting more desperate, so naturally I found myself considering some more extreme options. I had heard of a surgery called ETS that made it literally impossible to blush. It stopped up all of the blood vessels in your face so that blushing would never be a problem again. I thought that I had encountered my Holy Grail when, unfortunately, I started reading about the side effects. I could never play sports or exercise properly again because I had to watch my heart rate. The sweating on my face would be redistributed to other parts of my body, specifically my crotch. I would be at increased risk of heatstroke, even in mild weather. I hated blushing so much that I still considered this option, but then wisely deferred in favor of a more natural alternative. After all, surgery is irreversible.

I found myself spending hundreds of pounds on proposed herbal remedies for social disorders. While it seemed to work at first, nothing really ever helped me reliably. I still felt the anxiety and the emotions that led to blushing, and most of the time it was enough to overcome the effect of the herbal remedies. Frustrated, I threw my herbal remedies away and decided to try something that I had been dreading for a long, long time.

I know that therapy is generally well-accepted by society today, but my family had never been a subscriber to psychologists. In my family, therapy was a sign that you were crazy, that something was terribly wrong with you. But, even with this background ingrained in my mind,

I was desperate enough to try it. I realized that therapy was helpful in many ways. It taught me about the connection between my mind and my body, and to trace my past for reasons as to why I feel anxious today. But, while I sure learned a lot, I became impatient with the lack of substantial results. I was still blushing all of the time. I could not control the reaction my body had to social situations.

I began to think extremely negative things. I thought that, if therapy could not cure me, then no remedy on the planet could. I started blushing at the slightest hint of human contact. The grocery checkout counter became a huge ordeal. I was incapable of leading a normal life.

Then, one day, I made my breakthrough.

So, who exactly am I to tell you how to stop blushing? That's easy. I'm one of you. I've suffered all the extremes that this disorder can cause. I've spent lots and lots of money on unsuccessful and expensive treatments, only to find that they did nothing to help me. And I've come out alive, socially active, and happier than I could ever had imagined when I was a blusher.

You Are Not Alone

If you can relate to this story, then I have the best news in the world. The cure to blushing and social anxiety may be easier than *you ever thought possible.*

If you have social anxiety, then it's easy to feel like you're by yourself. Nobody cares about you. You're the only one in the world who has this problem, and there's nothing you can do about it. The world is like some kind of huge inside joke that you were purposely left out of.

It's only natural to feel this way. But an important step to recovery is recognizing that this is factually incorrect. Millions of people around the globe suffer from the same problem that you do. Some of them might be right next door. Some of them might be in your office, or you might see them as you pass them by in the grocery. We are everywhere.

This is an empowering thought for two reasons. One, it can go a long way to relieve the feelings of isolation that you get when you blush. You may feel like a strange person, but the fact that there are millions just like you means that, statistically speaking, you aren't that weird! Secondly, just as there are hordes of people just like you, there are many people who used to have the same problem but have overcome it! These people are not individuals of great ability or courage; rather, they are people just like you, who have experienced the same pain and conquered it. If I can, and if these people can, then you certainly can as well.

Who is This Book For?

There are many symptoms of social anxiety. If you find yourself blushing uncontrollably during social interactions, then this book is definitely for you. If you tend to assume that everyone is judging you whenever you walk into a room, then this book is for you. If your pulse races or your palms sweat whenever you deal with other people, then I can help you. If you know that you are a human being worth his carbon makeup and you are committed to living a happy life full of rich social relationships but just can't seem to find them, then look no further. If you know you have value but are unable to express this value because you act like a different person when you're nervous, then keep reading. Even if you're somewhat far along in your recovery process and you just want some tips and tricks to push you to that next level success, then this book is for you, too.

The Breakthrough!

Why am I so confident? Why am I so sure that this book can help people with any degree of social anxiety overcome their demons and start living the life they deserve? It's very simple. I have made the blushing breakthrough, and can share with you exactly how I did it. No medicines, no pills, no immediate cures or spiritual mumbo-jumbo. This system works, and I know, because it worked for me. I've told you my story, so I don't need to reiterate how much of a huge problem blushing was for me.

The Breakthrough program works because it doesn't offer an easy way out. I learned, in my journey, that people offering the easy way out are probably just after your money. Instead, this book is full of information and methods that will, over time, help you become the person that you want to be. This may disappoint you, but I assure you: there is no overnight cure. If this is what you want, then you will never recover. It takes hard work and dedication to these methods of recovery to make progress, and the progress will appear slow at first. But one day, you will wake up, take a look at yourself, and realize that your problem isn't nearly as bad as it used to be. You will feel more positive about yourself, which will give you the motivation and energy to challenge yourself even more. Soon, you will be using the past tense to refer to your condition.

There are four basic steps to this method. Each of these steps is covered thoroughly, so you won't be left hanging, wishing you had more information.

1. **Understanding:** Your problem may seem insurmountable. However, if you properly understand the biology and physiology of the issue, you will realize that it is anything but.
2. **Control Your Mind:** The mind is the most important organ in the body. You'll find some simple steps to slowly take control of your brain and tell it that you don't have a problem.
3. **Control Your Body:** You may think that blushing is mainly a mental problem, but did you know that the mind and the body are intricately connected? Here, you'll find some tips to use your body as a tool for overcoming blushing.
4. **The Next Level:** You should never stop learning and improving yourself. In here, you'll find some pointers for taking your newly-developed social skills to the next level and become the social butterfly you always wanted to be.

What are you waiting for? All of our time on this earth is precious. Stop wasting it by being anxious and blushing. Read this book, practice the steps and you'll be able to take advantage of your time sooner than you thought.

CHAPTER TWO

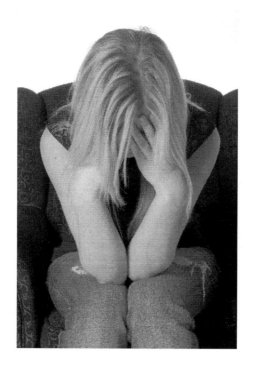

WHY DO WE BLUSH?

If you're reading this book with any intense level of interest, then the chances are that you've asked yourself this question many, many times. Why do we blush? What purpose does this useless thing have? Why is it ruining my ability to maintain normal social interactions?

You may be sick of asking yourself this question. After all, who cares exactly why we blush? *All I care about is how to make it stop!* The consequences of the problem are more embarrassing and more frustrating than the biological root of the problem, so you may feel like understanding how blushing works is trivial and unimportant, and a detour on your journey to achieving a blush-free lifestyle. Unfortunately, this could not be further from the truth.

Understanding what physically happens to your body when you blush is a crucial step in undermining the blushing thought process. Why? It's very simple. Humanity is conditioned to be afraid of what we do not understand. It's helped us survive countless situations in prehistoric times in which there literally was danger around every corner, and it helped our survival to fear what we didn't know was already safe.

This is the source of many of our modern-day problems. Our bodies are still programmed for pre-society, for living in the wild with predators and surviving off the land. There's no way for us to tell our bodies which evolutionary features we don't need anymore, except through the process of evolution, and it could literally take tens of thousands of years for our genes to realize that we don't use specific functions. No matter how hard we may yell at our bodies, they will still continue executing their natural functions, believing that they are keeping us alive.

There's good news, though! The reason that we humans have achieved such monumental things as a species is because we *have the most powerful minds on the globe!* We are able to control our minds and police our thoughts. If we understand why we do something biologically, it is possible for us to manipulate our brains in such a manner that we change our response to a certain stimulus! If you become a student of the science of blushing, you will be better equipped to find the mental tools and correct thought processes to stem the blushing attack before it occurs.

Another reason it's important to understand the science is blushing is to reduce our fear. Again, humans are afraid of what they do not understand. If you do not understand that blushing is a simple series of chemical reactions triggered by perfectly normal circumstances, then it's easy to focus on the consequences of blushing, and the toll it takes on your overall happiness. This can make blushing feel supernatural, like a dark spell that we've fallen under and we can't quite shake off. However, biologically speaking, this couldn't be further from the truth! If you were to understand your blushing, you would be marginally less afraid of it.

This is exactly the same idea that is in play when a child is afraid of the dark. Do you remember when you were young, and you were afraid of an open closet in the dark? Maybe not, but it's something we all experience. We can't see into the closet, so we have no idea what will come out of it, and this makes us afraid.

However, as we grow older and gain more knowledge, we come to recognize that something has to go *in* to the closet before something can come *out* of it. We realize that, as long as we don't see anything in the closet in the daytime, nothing can come out of it during the night. We understand the problem, and our fear dissipates.

You can influence your blushing in the same exact way. If you fear your blushing because you do not understand it, then it's easy to create a dark closet for blushing in your mind. However, if you understand your blushing, then you will see the bare closet for what it truly is: harmless!

Also, being terrified of blushing can make blushing attacks more intense, and will make you more likely to blush. If you understand that the first step to stemming the blushing tide is to cease being afraid of blushing, and the first step to cease being afraid of blushing is to understand blushing, then read onward.

Why Do We Blush?

The science of blushing is very complicated, and scientists do not yet fully understand what happens when we blush. This is because it is both *physiological* and *psychological,* and it's both *triggered* and *involuntary.* Our reaction to circumstances that make us blush is so complicated and difficult to comprehend because it involves so many different factors and reactions in our bodies.

There are many reasons why the human face turns red, or flushes. Many people turn red when they start drinking alcohol, or become sexually aroused, or angry. Although these situations have the exact same physical manifestation (a red face), these situations are different from blushing caused by embarrassment or anxiety because they are set in motion by a unique set of chemical reactions. Blushing from embarrassment, the problem that you face every day, is the only type of blushing caused by adrenaline. Thus, if you have a blushing problem, it isn't a physical problem: the human body has many reasons to turn red. People with blushing problems suffer from uncontrolled blushing as a result of adrenaline, and this specific type of blushing is completely triggered by your brain.

As I mentioned earlier, blushing from adrenaline is both a psychological and a physiological issue. It is psychological because it is triggered solely by an *emotional* stimulus. You don't start blushing because you get a certain set of physical or evolutionary triggers. You start blushing because of the way you feel. When you feel embarrassed or ashamed, the reaction begins.

After your brain perceives cues to feel embarrassed, it activates your "fight or flight" system, also known as your **sympathetic nervous system.** This system calls on your glands to release the hormone known as adrenaline, which is also triggered when your body perceives itself to be in grave danger from a predator and enables you to run away as fast as you possibly can. This shuts down or slows the digestive system so that more energy can be siphoned into the muscles. It also quickens your heart rate and your breathing so that you will be able to move quicker and react faster. It increases the size of your pupils so that you can take in more information and make quicker decisions.

What does any of this have to do with blushing? In order to further increase the performance potential of your body, adrenaline also activates a process called **vasodilation,** or the dilation of the blood vessels. This allows your body to pump oxygen-rich blood more efficiently to your muscles by increasing the amount of blood that can be delivered. The veins in your face react to stimulus from a chemical transmitter called the **adenylyl cyclase**, which prompts the veins to dilate. This creates more localized blood flow in your face, which causes the reddish tint you have come to know so well.

If adrenaline makes your veins in your face dilate, then why exactly does your entire body not turn red as well? This is the facet of blushing that scientists do not fully understand. Veins elsewhere in the body are not responsive to adrenaline; when adrenaline is activated, they do nothing differently. For some reason, adrenaline only dilates the veins in your face. The capillaries and other blood vessels are affected by adrenaline universally, but veins are usually not responsive. The veins in your face, however, light up like a Christmas tree, causing you to blush. This phenomenon, along with the fact that blushing is an emotionally-triggered mechanism, has led scientists to believe that there may be an evolutionary reason in play.

The Evolutionary Reason behind Blushing

If there isn't a specific, logical anatomical reason behind blushing, then there must be some reason why our bodies felt the need to develop the act of blushing as we evolved. But what could it be? It's somewhat hard to think of a good reason why evolution would dictate us to get red in the face when we feel embarrassed. Certainly predators do not care if we are embarrassed. There must be some reason why it helps our survival to show embarrassment on our faces. There's no concrete way to figure this out, but scientists have some theories.

Dr. Ray Crozier, a leading psychologist at the University of East Anglia, theorizes that humans blush as a way of automatically apologizing for social mistakes. Humans are inertly social creatures, and we are programmed with many tools (such as emotions like guilt, empathy, etc.) that assist us in functioning as a society. Blushing may just be another tool that enables more efficient social communication. If we blush whenever we make a mistake or make someone feel bad, we feel embarrassed as a result, and we wear it on our face as punishment. This also lets the offended party know that we feel bad, which is an important step in establishing empathy. "A prerequisite for embarrassment is to be able to feel how others feel -- you have to be empathetic, intelligent to the social situation" Crozier says. If we show our embarrassment on our faces, this is an unmistakable social cue that the offending party is empathic with the anger that he or she has caused, and is truly sorry for whatever offense they have committed because they can imagine themselves in the same situation. In this theory, blushing can lower the risk of a violent or elevated incident because the offender expresses automatic remorse through blushing.

Some theorists take this idea even further, to the most basic pre-historic core of our being. Before the advent of civilized society, something as much as a slight insult could lead to an all-out tribal war. If one of our prehistoric brethren were to accidentally insult a leader of a pack or tribe, it could easily get him stabbed or killed. However, blushing kicks in as a way of automatically expressing submission to the aggressor, making them less likely to attack in response.

Think about a master/dog relationship. If the master is displeased with his dog because it has eaten a meal off of the table, a common response would be to threaten to hit the dog, or punish it physically. The dog, sensing this anger, will sit down and look sad or roll over on its back to express submission. Biologically speaking, unless you're a sociopath, you will have a much harder time summoning the will to hit the dog after it shows you that it is not challenging your anger.

The same principle can be applied to humans. ==If we automatically show our remorse and submission, then the person we have offended is less likely to take harmful physical==

action. In this way, blushing is a tool designed to help societies function more smoothly by discouraging acts of man-on-man violence due to insult and social faux pass.

If you have a blushing problem, then the root of that problem lies in the fact that your brain is programmed to show submission, even when such a display of submission is completely unnecessary, biologically unattractive, and fully counterproductive. Why does your brain feel the need to constantly be showing submission to others? Because you have an anxiety problem.

Blushing, in fact, is simply a physical symptom of social anxiety disorder. Social anxiety disorder is characterized by excessive feelings of worry that others are judging you or don't like you. Because we are such social creatures by nature, if we feel emotionally that people do not like us, then our brains' evolutionary response would be to activate the blushing mechanism out of self-defense. Remember, our instincts still think that we can be hurt or killed from a social insult (they don't take the law into account,) so if you worry excessively about social situations, you will constantly be putting your brain on alert to activate the "fight or flight" system and release adrenaline. If you find yourself constantly blushing at even the most minor of social circumstances, your anxious brain is misinterpreting these interactions as potentially offensive to the other person, and is activating the blushing mechanism to apologize for any possible offense.

This is both the blessing and the curse of social anxiety: **it's all in your head.** You feel that even the most ordinary of circumstances can put you at risk for messing up, acting nervous, or being judged, but this **isn't even close to the reality.** People successfully interact with others every day; it's part of our DNA. It's not that you were born with some kind of social deformity. You are afraid of what other people think of you, so you, in turn, reduce your ability to perform socially. It's a cruel cycle, and a self-fulfilling prophecy, but the good news is that *there's absolutely nothing wrong with you!* It's just a trick your brain is playing on you, based solely on your past experiences. While getting your brain out of this negative loop can certainly be tricky, it's certainly far from impossible, and is much easier than you think. While different things work to various degrees on different people, the exercises and tools within this book should give you a wide range of options, so you can select what methods make you feel the best.

For many people, simply understanding the problem goes a long way to recovery. Picture your anxiety as an insurmountable mountain. There doesn't seem to be any way up, and it doesn't feel like there's any way you'll ever get over it. But now that you understand why you act the way that you do, a giant light shines on the mountain, and you can see everything clearly. Turns out, there was a handy set of stairs winding all the way to the top and back down on the other side! You just couldn't find the stairs before because you were searching around in the dark. The mountain is still in front of you, and it's still yours to climb, but at least you know for sure that there's a way to get over it.

The Top Nine Blush-Inducing Feelings

So you know what makes you blush from a biological and evolutionary perspective, but that doesn't relate specifically to your life. You can't see the veins dilating or the adrenaline moving through your system, but you do see what happens when people see you become a blushing mess. What kinds of feelings induce your brain to activate the blushing mechanism?

Like everything in this book, the answer depends on the specific person. Some people are more sensitive to certain circumstances, while other people will blush at everything. Still, we can identify the top nine reasons why people start blushing from a social-situational perspective. You will definitely be familiar with some of these and may be able to relate to all of them, but regardless of how many of these sound familiar, if you start to understand what kind of feelings make you start blushing, you'll be better equipped to stop it. At the end of this book, we'll go back through these nine emotions and feelings and note how you've learned to combat them.

1. **Shame:** This is the purest form of blushing in an evolutionary sense. You are embarrassed by something you've done or something you've said, and can turn as red as a tomato. This is completely normal. Most people blush when they are ashamed of something they did. Whether you put your foot in your mouth or said the wrong thing at the wrong time, or accidentally tripped someone.

2. **Humiliation:** When someone ridicules you or insults you in a public place, or in front of your friends, then you can't help but feel a little humiliated. The fact that someone called attention to one of your faults can be embarrassing, and can trigger a blushing reaction.

3. **Shyness:** People with social anxiety often struggle with finding things to say in front of people that they don't know very well. While it's normal to be more socially conscious while around new people, it's not healthy or productive to shrivel up into a corner and close your mouth. The simple presence of people that you aren't familiar with can lead you to thinking that they are judging you, and can cause you to blush.

4. **Gratitude:** If someone does something that really helps you out, you will feel grateful, and want to express this to the other person. Unfortunately, people with social anxiety can be unsure of how to express this emotion tactfully and effectively, and it can cause them to become embarrassed.

5. **Love or Intense Emotionality:** This is very similar to gratitude. People with social anxiety feel these emotions on the same level that normal people do, but get nervous when they feel like they need to express that emotion. They feel that they will come off as awkward, and will not

express how they are feeling clearly, causing them to blush.

6. **Recognition:** This is a positive emotion that can easily set off a blushing attack. Even though you're being recognized for something you've done well, your fear of having attention called to yourself can override what pride results from the recognition. You may feel that you don't know how to act or what to say when all eyes are on you.

7. **Exposure:** This is very similar to Recognition. If you are placed in front of a large group of people whose attention is entirely fixed on you (say you are making a public speech or are being recorded on camera), the pressure to make a good impression on so many people may cause you to become embarrassed.

8. **Pressure:** If you have an important date or business meeting where you know that you need to impress people in order to reap great rewards, the possibility of failing and not achieving what you want can make you nervous, which can

cause you to become anxious. This is particularly frustrating, because you actually lower your chances of success when you aren't relaxed.

9. **Anticipation:** The mere expectation of being put under any of the situations above can cause you to blush. This will certainly guarantee a blushing attack when the situation actually occurs.

Remember these nine emotional triggers! At the end of this book, we will re-visit this list and discuss how you have conquered these seemingly insurmountable emotional obstacles.

You should now have a pretty good idea of why you blush. This may seem kind of arbitrary, but it is an important tool and the foundation for any future healing. In the next chapter, we will discuss mental techniques that you can use to reduce your blushing and regain control over your life.

CHAPTER THREE

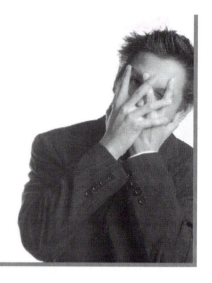

CONTROL YOUR MIND

As you well know by now, the mind is the most powerful organ in the human body. The way that you think about things can determine your reactions, your outlook on life, your happiness, and even your physical health. It's patently obvious, then, that the number one key to controlling your blushing problem is to control your mind. There are many ways to do this, and this chapter is loaded with exercises, techniques, and tricks that will help you gain control of this organ and direct it to do exactly what you want it to do.

People with anxiety disorders let their minds control them. They base their reactions and behaviors on things that they have experienced and seen in the past, and it controls their future. But think about this: *the past is the past!* If you wanted to live the rest of your life based on the past, then you have no future to look forward to whatsoever!

The brain is a muscle. If you wanted to raise your arm, all you would need to do is tell your brain to send the correct electrical signals to your muscles and they would follow your command. The same is true for your mind: you just need to learn how to control it. How do you achieve this?

Well, how would you achieve better control over a muscle? You would probably go to the gym and work out with weights and aerobics until you felt that you had a better understanding of how the muscle worked and what you could do to strengthen it. The same concept applies to the mind. If you exercise your mind and practice doing certain things, then your mind will get into shape, and you will be able to control it! It won't happen overnight (you don't expect to go to the gym once and wake up the next day with the body of an athlete), but if you work at it, you will put your blushing days behind you.

After we review some common pitfalls that the average blusher encounters in his or her journey, we can start reviewing some exercises that will help you put yourself into the correct frame of mind.

The Biggest Mistake You're Probably Already Making

If you've had problems with social anxiety and blushing for an extended period of time, chances are that you try to devote an inordinate amount of your time attempting to "tackle" this problem. You've probably seen therapists and taken medications. Every time the problem rears its ugly head, you probably think something like "I'm not going to let my problem affect me this time. I'm going to beat it." You probably spend a lot of time thinking about the fact that you have a problem, and spend your time trying to address it. If this is what you do (and if you still have a blushing problem, you definitely do) then you are making one of the biggest mistakes you could possibly be making when it comes to controlling your blushing problem:

YOU THINK THAT YOU HAVE A PROBLEM.

You may think to yourself, "Well, I obviously have a problem. I can't talk to people successfully, and I can't even leave the house without having a blushing episode."

But there's something you need to understand. You do not feel this way because you have a medical disorder. You cannot go to the doctor and get an x-ray and have the doctor point out the root of the problem. You are not deformed.

This is what happened to you: somewhere along the line, something happened to you that made you feel like you were a socially incompetent, isolated pariah of a person. Then, you became so afraid of it happening again that you decided that you had a problem, instead of giving it another shot.

Therefore, the only thing that separates you from a normal person is undoing or forgetting the damage of the past. You don't have a problem; **you have a mental roadblock that can be easily taken down.**

If you think of yourself as having a problem, you are feeling sorry for yourself. You are making excuses for not taking action by categorizing yourself as "troubled" and making it seem like you are the victim of some unfortunate circumstance. **STOP FEELING SORRY FOR YOURSELF, NOW.** The sooner you change the way that you look at your situation, the sooner that you will have power over it. This is fact.

The problem with self-pity is that it's usually the only thing sustaining your state of mind. Every time a social situation occurs, you've been thinking about the fact that you have a problem so often that it comes to mind right away. You remind yourself, before and during the situation, that you have a problem, and that you are struggling with a disease. This serves as a self-fulfilling prophecy. Because you are thinking of the situation in terms of your alleged "problem", your actions and your physiology respond accordingly, and you begin to blush. You then leave that situation even more certain that you have a problem, and you wallow in self-despair.

The solution to this problem is remarkably simple. You need to practice thinking differently. After two weeks of practice, your mindset will have already changed, and you will be ready to try more advanced things.

Every day, right when you get out of bed, grab a sheet of paper and write "I am a completely normal person. There is nothing at all wrong with me. I do not have a problem. I can interact with people just as well as anybody else." Then, think of ten things that you think other people would like about you. No matter who you are, you have likeable characteristics. List these in bullet points below the statement, and keep this line of thought in your head as you go through your day. At the end of the day, throw this paper out, tear it up and get rid of it. The next day, repeat the same process. Alter your mantra however you see fit, and keep adding things to your list.

This may seem very stupid and simple, but the fact is that repetition is a great way to alter your brain chemistry. It won't work right away, and you may have doubts and want to quit, but the fact is that if you keep doing it every day, slowly your brain will start to believe what you are writing, and you will notice that you think more positively about yourself. Don't just look at the same list every day; studies have proven that writing something ingrains it in your mind more effectively than simply reading something. In a way, you are doing push-ups for your mind: small little exercises that make no big difference when looked at individually but have great effect when done constantly, over a long period of time.

The Three Pre-Programmed Mental Faults of Blushers

During my own recovery time, I noticed that I had three principle mental faults that I kept falling back on. Every time I had an episode, I would keep thinking along these three faulty lines, and they went a long way to keep me down. After my recovery, as I began to help others cope with their blushing problems, I began to notice these exact same patterns in the thoughts of others as well.

If you're like I was, then you probably have these faults as well. The bad news is that these mental faults are deeply ingrained in your mind because you've been practicing them for a long time. The good news, on the other hand, is that there's a really simple fix. **These faults are exactly that: faults!** These are errors in thinking. They aren't based on fact, or anything tangible. The solution is simple. Examine your thoughts more carefully the next time you have an episode, and try to spot these underlying errors. If you recognize them as incorrect, then you rob them of all of their power over you.

1. **You think you are different:** Wrong! Can you show me on an x-ray or a cat scan what makes you different? Do you have a third arm sticking out of your body somewhere? Do you have an inoperable tumor on your brain that clogs your social cognitive function? No. You do not. The only thing that makes you different from everyone else is that you've managed to psych yourself out and get into some bad mental habits. That's it.

2. **You think other people can spot your issues just by looking at you:** Wrong! You spend so much time inside of your head, contemplating your problem that you think that someone can tell what's wrong with you just by looking at you. The truth is that people have no idea what you're going through. If you're having a blushing fit, then yes, people will get an idea. But, before you start blushing, you look like a perfectly normal, healthy person who other people can appreciate and respect. Most people are too worried about what you think of them to think about what they think of you anyway

3. **You can't imagine an end to your problem:** Wrong! Of course you can't! Our minds actually have very poor imaginations. They have a lot of trouble picturing what things will be like if we felt differently because they base their future predictions on past experiences, which is the only thing that they can rely on. Just because you can't imagine how things would be without

your issues doesn't mean it's impossible. That's just natural! You need to work on training your mind to think in a way that you've never thought before, and it will appear obvious to you after you've arrived at your mental destination.

Every time you have an attack, you will find yourself thinking along one of these three lines (or all three!) Simply recognize that these are logical fallacies and re-direct your mind along more positive lines, using…

Positive Feedback Loops

Blushers and people with social anxiety naturally have low self-esteem. We are surrounded with motivational images that tell us not to care what people think about us, but these were invariably written by people with friends. The reason we have survived and flourished as a species up to this point is because we are naturally programmed to be social creatures. That's right, I said it: **You're supposed to care what other people think about you.** You just can't care about what *everyone* thinks about you, because what one person likes, another person may find completely loathsome.

It's only logical, then, that people with low-self esteem from a lack of human validation and contact tend to think very negative thought patterns. Even when you aren't nervous or blushing, you will find yourself criticizing yourself too harshly, or always looking at the worst side of people or events. You probably have a pessimistic outlook, and feel that all of your hopes are silly delusions. You have thought this way for so long that you see it as the way the world works, rather than your point of view.

Here's an interesting fact: **"the way the world works" is entirely up to you.** A pretty fair share of negative and positive things happen every single day; you just have the tendency to only notice the negative ones. If you took the time to notice all of the positive things that happen to you on a daily basis, you will find that they are just as common as the negative ones. You just never bothered paying any attention!

This is where creating a "positive feedback loop" comes in to play. There are three easy steps to implementing a more positive outlook in your life. The more you practice them and integrate them into your daily routine, the more noticeably sunny your outlook will become. The old saying "Good things happen to positive people" is completely true, not because positive people have better luck but because they have the positive energy and the hope to take advantage of opportunities as they arise. A negative person may simply disregard a possible opening as a long shot and not even bother trying. They might be passing up on a huge chance to succeed!

1. **Congratulate yourself for everything you do correctly:** People with blushing issues tend to be rough on themselves when they have an episode or when they do something wrong. They completely forget to congratulate themselves when they do something well! No feat is too small to qualify for laudation. You've

been writing positive thoughts every morning for a week? Reward yourself. You did something nice for a neighbor or co-worker for no personal reward? Savor your victory! Did you complete a project at work to the best of your ability? Buy yourself an ice cream. You deserve it.

2. **Think about failure differently:** Every time something doesn't quite go your way, it's easy to be tough on yourself and consider it a total failure. The error with this line of thinking is that you assume that you always have to succeed in order to be a success. This is false. Even the most successful people fail, and fail constantly, in order to eventually achieve success. You should be interpreting each failure as a learning experience, as a chance to grow through objectively observing your mistakes and making corrections for your next try. You'll find that not only will you get closer and closer to success, but also you'll start to think about yourself in a more positive light.

3. **Interpret other people through a positive lens:** If you suffer from severe social anxiety or blushing, then chances are you see the worst in people. Say co-worker Tom came by and dropped off a stapler that he had borrowed. You would probably think about what a miserable person Tom was for returning it so late, or how lazy he was for not having a stapler of his own. This is counterproductive thinking! Instead, thank Tom and think about what a nice guy Tom was for returning your stapler without you having to go and get it back yourself. Absolutely, absolutely avoid jealousy at all costs. Instead, channel those intense feelings into effort, and try to get what you want so that you don't have to feel jealous. If you dislike people because you pre-empt their judgment of you with your judgment of them, then people will definitely not like you and your unfriendly vibes. Give everyone the benefit of the doubt, and they will appreciate it and return the favor down the road.

You shouldn't stop here, either! Every time a senseless negative thought enters your mind, banish it and replace it with a positive thought. You won't be making things up, just looking at the world a little differently. In time, you will start to gain more self-respect, which will make a huge difference when it comes to attempting…

The Seven Keys to Reprogramming your Brain

Now that you've got some practice thinking more positively about yourself and discarding negative and self-defeating thoughts, it's time to turn your attention to the actual reprogramming of your brain. Remember, there isn't anything wrong with you; your brain is just incorrectly programmed to have an irrational fear of social embarrassment.

I looked back at the time in which I was recovering from my own social issues, and traced the seven behavior patterns that had the most effect on changing the way I view myself and my interactions with other people. I've listed them here below. Again, you can't be out to prove this system wrong. You have to actively, constantly be working on controlling your thoughts and following these steps, and you will notice improvement very quickly. If you skeptically fight this process, then it won't matter how many books you read; you will always reflect your negative attitude in how you compose yourself and how you interact with other people.

1. **Police Your Thoughts:** Do NOT allow yourself to think about your condition. Has contemplating your "problem" ever led you to any successes, or has it only led to more thinking and circular logic? No matter how often you try to rationalize or "figure out" your phobias, this will do nothing productive and actually keep them in place. In your mind, you do not have a problem. It may still surface sometimes during episodes, but you cannot allow yourself to think about it. Read a book, watch a film, do anything, but DO NOT THINK ABOUT IT.

2. **Meditate:** We will cover basic instructions on how to do this in the next chapter, but meditation is in an invaluable mental tool as well as a physical relaxant. When you learn to meditate, you learn to clear your mind of all thoughts and be at peace. Learning how to quickly empty your mind is a precious tool when negative and anxious thoughts start building up right before a social interaction.

3. **Exercise:** Again, this will be covered more thoroughly in the next chapter, but exercise releases natural relaxants in your body called endorphins that promote a sense of well-being. If you exercise constantly, you will find that it will become harder and harder to blush, as the presence of the endorphins makes it more difficult for negative thoughts to take hold.

4. **Force Yourself to Confront Your Fear:** This is quite possibly the most productive and important step in this list. If you find yourself blushing at every single social interaction, you will become tempted to do as I did. If you remember, what I

did was hole myself up in my apartment, feeling sorry for myself, avoiding personal contact at all costs. This is the *worst thing you can possibly do to yourself!* Instead, you need to do the exact opposite and confront your fear head-on. Design a program for yourself in which you force yourself to have a simple social interaction with a stranger every single day, even if it terrifies you and makes you sick in your stomach. This way, you are reprogramming your brain to stop being afraid of other people. Remember, your mind is afraid of social interaction because of things that happened in your past. What you need to do is show your mind that interacting with your fellow man simply **isn't that bad.** You may be absolutely terrified the first couple times, but after you practice swallowing your fear and talking to people (even if you turn into a total blushing mess), your brain will start to understand the process better, and you will become less afraid of it. Think about when you learned to ride a bicycle or swim. Do you remember how scared you were the first few times you tried it? Most people are terrified out of their minds. Now, how do you feel about these activities today? You can probably perform these activities without even paying much attention to them, as an afterthought. The same principle can be applied to social interactions. You must **demystify** and **normalize** social interactions, and make them routine to your mind, and the only way to do this is through practice. Remember that the only goal is to practice and normalize, not achieve results. Results come later. Even if you make a total fool out of yourself and walk away feeling poorly, you have taken a small step towards confronting your fear. If you keep it up, the rest will come naturally.

5. **Never Panic:** Every time you embarrass yourself through a blushing episode, the easiest thing to do is to go home and cry. You must adjust this behavior pattern. View each failure as a learning experience on your journey to recovery instead of reinforcing your old thoughts. If you

find that you become less depressed after every episode, you will fear having an episode a lot less.

6. **Always Adjust:** This book is a great place to start, but everybody's journey is different. I would be a fool or a liar if I told you I had a one-size-fits-all solution to blushing. Always be self-observant, and try to improve your mental methods and your techniques after every failure and after every success. If you constantly adjust your recovery method, you will find the best one that works for you in no time.

7. **Keep a Thought Log:** Grab a sheet of paper and divide it into two halves, one for negative thoughts and one for positive thoughts. Record on this piece of paper what kind of thoughts made you feel like you were a healthy, socially active person. Then, on the other side, record thoughts that led up to a blushing attack or a fit of social phobia. Negative feelings and anxiety usually snowball from insignificant and minor-seeming thoughts. If you learn to never repeat

the thoughts on the negative side of the column and replace those thoughts with those on the positive side of the column, then you will eliminate the "seed thought" that got you worried or embarrassed in the first place, and your fears will have nothing to build on.

What to Do During an Attack

Even if you focus your every effort on becoming a more positive and social person, you will still occasionally have blushing attacks, especially in the first couple months. While these attacks will soon be a thing of the past, you need to learn how to control these attacks when they do happen. If you manage to stop an attack in the process, you will have taken a large step in the process of eliminating your dread and fear of attacks occurring again in the future. Stopping an attack while it's happening is a sign of progress to even the most skeptical and frustrated blushers. This method will take some practice, but these are the three steps I used whenever I felt an attack coming. After seven or eight tries, I was able to stop my blushing episodes in their tracks consistently, within thirty seconds.

1. **Tunnel-Vision Yourself:** If you feel an episode coming on, immediately focus all of your attention on something unrelated to your issue. If you're out at a restaurant, focus a single waiter across the room, or the way that the napkin is folded, or the font that the menu is printed in. You must re-route your thoughts away from the episode by legitimately distracting yourself from it. Pick something that interests you, or change the conversation to something that you can focus on, and do not think about anything else. If you allow your mind to wander, you will invariably remind yourself that you are blushing, and the attack will continue. Do NOT acknowledge that the issue exists by stepping out to the bathroom, or exist it shall.
2. **Regulate your Breathing:** If you pay attention, you will find that your pulse will quicken and your breaths will become short during an episode.

Oxygen is a natural relaxant, and can keep your body temperature from rising and your heart from racing. Subtly start to take deep, long breaths, without calling attention to yourself. This will do its part to physically keep you calm.

3. **Engage in your Surroundings:** Falling silent and staring at the floor has the exact same effect as thinking about your problem. You need to convince yourself that nothing bad is happening. Try to up the level of conversation, and keep participating, no matter how red you get. If you become self-conscious and fall silent, then you will have an episode, and that will be the end of the night.

The mind is your greatest enemy when trying to overcome blushing and social anxiety. In order to truly defeat your issue, you will have to reprogram it to become your best friend. If you practice the exercises and methods I've listed in this chapter diligently and hopefully, then you will begin to see results. Trust me, if I did it (and I did), then you can too.

CHAPTER FOUR

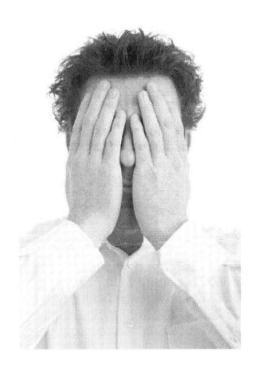

CONTROL YOUR BODY

One common mistake that you may be making when trying to control your blushing or social anxiety problem is you are neglecting to consider your body and your physical health. It may seem somewhat strange to consider your body when trying to deal with an issue that is clearly mental. After all, the blushing situation is in your head, right? Isn't that what we've been covering for the last two chapters? So what you put in to your body and the things you do with it have nothing to do with blushing, right?

Wrong. Doctors and scientists all over the globe have recognized the mind-body connection for well over two decades now. There is incontrovertible evidence that your mental health has an effect on your physical health, and vice versa. People who have serious illnesses are more likely to survive and recover if they do not give up mentally and stay positive. The reverse applies to mental illnesses.

Why? It's simple. We humans may think that when we feel down or depressed, something is wrong emotionally or mentally and there's nothing we can concretely do about it. This just isn't the case in reality, though. Moods, feelings, and thoughts can all be caused by physical conditions. Why do you think people get grumpy when they're really hungry?

Our physical condition strongly influences our emotional condition. A balanced diet can go a long way to promote good physical feelings of health, which are proven to reduce mental stress. Exercise releases endorphins, which serve as a natural drug and promote happiness and feelings of well-being (which counteract your negative emotional attitudes.) Certain herbal remedies can go a long way to helping us relax and keeping us calm. If we are physically relaxed, through meditation or stretching exercises, then it is much easier to become mentally relaxed.

What does all of this mean? It means that, in order to control your social anxiety or your blushing problem, you must learn to control your body and put it in the best shape for recovery. I neglected this part of my treatment for a long time, and I felt the difference almost immediately once I integrated physical exercise into my routine. I felt more confident, generally healthier, and had more energy and motivation to tackle the mental exercises I listed in the previous chapter. In this chapter, I'll give you some basic hints on how to implement better physical health into your life that will improve your chances of overcoming this problem and living the life you've always dreamed about.

Fix your Diet

Imagine how you feel after you've eaten two bacon cheeseburgers, a large fry, and a milkshake. Do you feel energetic and ready to tackle the challenges of the day? Or do you feel like you want to plant yourself on the couch and never move again? What we eat has a huge amount of influence over how much energy we have and how we feel emotionally. You cannot expect to have the energy and the motivation to conquer your blushing situation if you eat an unhealthy diet. In fact, a poor diet can directly lead to depression and anxiety, even if you don't have a problem! So imagine how much harder you are making it on yourself by eating poorly.

The Catch-22

This seems easy enough, right? Nobody likes feeling bad emotionally, so if you simply avoid poor diet, then you will make it easier on yourself.

But there's a problem. When we feel depressed, anxious, or unmotivated, we have a hard time finding the motivation to eat correctly. We may feel like the only thing that we enjoy is food, and choose the best-tasting foods that are high in fat instead of smarter choices. We may feel like we have no time, and stick to our greasy fast-food diet choices instead of making more educated ones. We may feel like our problems are unsolvable, and that there's just no point in paying attention to our diets.

This can lead to an uncomfortable Catch-22. If we eat better, then we will feel better emotionally. However, because we don't feel good emotionally, we aren't inclined to fix our diets!

Look at it this way: you can't willingly just turn off your social anxiety. It takes practice, mental reprogramming, and the formation of new habits. So what can we change immediately? Our diets! Our brains tend to direct our thoughts to follow our behaviors. If you change the behavior (which you have control over), then the thoughts (which are harder to control) will follow! One great way to change your behavior is to improve your diet in the following ways:

1. **Avoid Processed Foods:** It may be mighty tempting to grab that TV dinner or that frozen pizza. It's cheaper and less time consuming than cooking, right? Well, the truth is, the more foods you eat that are loaded with chemicals, preservatives, and coloring agents, the less healthy you are going to feel. We aren't supposed to eat the stuff that we make in a lab, we're supposed to eat the stuff that we find in

nature! Avoid the over-processed snack cakes and preserved pre-made foods and stick to fresh meats, fruits, and vegetables when designing your diet.

2. **Avoid Refined Sugar and Flour:** This is one thing that you may not be used to doing. After all, refined white sugars and flours are everywhere, in many of our favorite foods. However, more and more studies are coming out that suggest that refined white sugar and flour is a leading cause of some forms of cancer and other serious diseases. Eating these foods is equivalent to slowly (very slowly) poisoning yourself. These foods will not give your body the fresh, energetic attitude that you will need to conquer your blushing. Opt for whole-grain breads and snacks instead of those using white flour, and check the sugar content of everything you eat. Do NOT drink sodas or artificial juices, as these are a great way to raise your anxiety levels and your daily sugar intake without realizing it! We often only pay attention to what we eat, not what we

drink. Avoid foods with over 30g of sugar per serving, and locate things made with cane sugar or natural syrups instead of white sugar. Try sweetening your baked goods with agave or honey instead of cups and cups of nasty, artificially-made sweeteners. They will still taste great, and you will feel much healthier.

3. **Avoid Caffeine:** Many people just can't seem to functions in the mornings unless they get their requisite cup of coffee or have an energy drink. Some people feel the need to take these products every single day! If you're a normal person (without an anxiety disorder), then occasional caffeine isn't bad, but having a daily dose just isn't good for you. If you're a person with anxiety, then the stimulant can make you jittery, feel nervous for no reason, and can make you easily startled, irritable, or high-strung. Stimulants just don't work for people with anxiety disorders; it amounts to shooting yourself in the foot. Get over it, and drop the coffee from your morning routine. If you feel like you still need

that extra push, then you can take a vitamin B-12 supplement that won't make you crash or feel jittery while still perking you up.

4. **Avoid Foods that are High in Fat:** That bacon double cheeseburger may look mighty tasty, but the fact is that your metabolism will grind to a halt trying to process all of that fat. Avoid red meats, excessive amounts of cheese, and pork products. Try to eliminate foods that are rich in butter or other dairy products. Check the label of every food you eat, and make sure that it is low in calories from fat and saturated fats, which are much more damaging than natural fats. Absolutely avoid anything with trans-fats, as these can clog your arteries and lead to heart disease. Try to get your daily fat from natural foods such as olives, peanuts, and oils, and not from greasy foods. Foods that are high in unhealthy fats will give your body a slow, weighed-down feeling that will hurt your motivation to try new things and to exercise, and you will find yourself sitting on the couch more

often than not, wasting yet another day not tackling your blushing problem.

5. **Eat Organic Foods:** Organic foods are defined by those that are completely natural in the ingredient list and in their processing methods. They do not contain artificial or chemical ingredients, and are not treated by means that use chemical purifiers or unnatural preservation agents. These foods are essentially in the same condition as they are found in nature. Eating a diet that is rich in organic foods cuts down the amount of chemicals you put into your body, and can help promote a better sense of well-being, which can go a long way to helping you gather the strength to take the mental and tangible steps to reducing your social anxiety.

6. **Eat a Diet Rich in Fruits and Vegetables:** If you be sure to get four to five servings of fruits and vegetables every single day, you will find that you feel much more energetic, less weighed-down, and your metabolism will function much better. This may seem like cliché advice that you

have been receiving your entire life, but the fact is that eating a diet rich in fruits and vegetables promotes good health and puts that extra spring in your step. If you have a severe blushing problem, you know that you will take whatever resources you can get.

7. **Eat Four to Five Times per Day:** With your busy schedule, it may seem easier to simply put off eating until you have the time to consume one giant meal near the end of the day. Unfortunately, this is really bad for your health for several reasons. One, putting off eating robs your body of energy that it needs to function at its highest level, and your concentration and energy levels will suffer immensely as a result. Secondly, your metabolism will not be able to process the massive amount of food that you consume during this single meal, and you will experience a lazy, sedated feeling that will prevent you from feeling good and meeting your objectives as your body redirects energy away from other functions to attempt to digest

the food. Thirdly, this can lead to weight gain, which can lower your self-esteem and your energy levels. Eat a big breakfast, and eat often throughout the day, at least four or five times, to ensure that you are giving your body the fuel that it needs.

8. **Take Vitamin and Mineral Supplements:** Vitamins and minerals are essential to proper bodily function. If you eat a diet that is rich in raw green vegetables or fruits, then you are probably already getting the amount that you need. If, however, you are particularly averse to these foods, then one solution is to take a vitamin and mineral supplement every day. These can boost your energy and help your concentration, and make you less likely to feel downtrodden or fatigued.

Diet is one of the most important things you can change when trying to overcome your blushing issues! Even after you overcome your situation (which you will), your new diet will ensure that you have the most energy possible and will help you live a longer and more complete life, so there's simply no reason to procrastinate on this. Improving your diet can even save you money! If you eat out all of the time, you are probably spending more money than you need to on your food budget. Go to the grocery store, plan your meals, and follow the above tips to ensure you are getting the most benefits from your food.

Five Easy Physical Exercises

Healthy, frequent rigorous exercise is another great way to improve your general mood and your physical condition. Exercise releases endorphins, which promote feelings of well-being, and can provide you with more energy. It can also help you sleep better at night, which is an absolutely crucial facet of cultivating a healthy lifestyle (and one that can give you the drive you need to overcome blushing.) Any type of exercise is helpful, but there are five exercises you can do without spending a dime at a gym or needing to drive to any off-site facility. You can also employ the services of a personal trainer to maximize your results if this is within your budget.

1. **Jogging:** This is one of the most common physical exercises for a good reason. It's easy, you can do it anywhere, and anyone can do it. Remember, jogging and running is very difficult if you aren't in good shape, so start slowly and build up a regimen. You don't need to be an endurance runner or a sprinter right away; you just need to get enough activity to release endorphins and burn calories. Start by setting a reasonable goal that you know you can meet (i.e. half a mile per day) and then diligently build on that number as you become acclimated to the exercise. Don't become complacent in your distance, or you will stop improving. Continue to push yourself within reason, and you will begin to notice results in your body shape, energy levels, and even general positivity.

2. **Walking:** If you don't have the time in your day to jog around the neighborhood, then you can

integrate physical activity into your daily routine through choosing to walk to more places. Instead of driving to work or to a friend's house, try walking or biking. Find excuses to use your legs instead of your car on a daily basis, and you will see how this minor adjustment can yield some serious results.

3. **Squats:** This is a household exercise you can do at any time. It goes a long way to strengthen your legs and your lower body, which promotes circulation and improves your energy levels. This exercise can be done with or without the use of weights, but you want to make sure that you are giving your legs a decent workout. If it feels too easy, it probably is, so push yourself. If you don't know how to do this exercise, simply type the word "squats" into your favorite search engine for a plethora of results and helpful how-to websites.

4. **Push-ups:** This exercise is a great way to work out your chest (pectoral muscles) and arms (biceps and triceps muscles), as well as some areas of

your back and your abdominal core. It can also go a long way to help your posture, which is another critical element of maintaining feelings of well-being. Make sure that you are using the proper technique, as exercises that are performed incorrectly do you no good and can even be harmful. Again, consult the internet or a fitness professional if you need guidance on how to perform this simple exercise.

5. **Sit-Ups:** These are a great way to work your abs and your core. A strong core region is absolutely essential to promoting fitness, as this is the area where fat tends to build up the quickest. Sit-ups also burn calories and release endorphins, and they're easy to do and can be done anywhere at any time.

If you successfully integrate these simple exercises into your daily routine, you will find yourself a more physically able, confident, and energetic person. These may not seem to relate to your social anxiety or blushing problem directly, but, as we discussed before, maintaining a healthy physical body makes the arduous process of conquering your blushing more manageable, and it can be the only difference between a successful recovery and more weeks and months wasted by locking yourself away from the rest of the world.

Posture and Massage

Two often-overlooked elements that will help you overcome your fear of social interaction are your posture and a massage regimen. Anxiety tends to cause muscle tension, which causes discomfort, headaches, poor spinal integrity, and can lead to major health problems as you get older. All of these can be very distracting when trying to focus on overcoming your blushing issue, and can lead you to feel like you are stuck with this problem permanently. The fact is that isn't the case! There are some very simple things you can do to improve your posture and release tension in your muscles that will help you become a more relaxed person.

One, be aware of your posture at all times. Your spine should be as straight as possible. If you work at a computer, be sure to sit up completely straight. Get a chair that makes this comfortable if you need to. Do not slouch or constantly bend your neck to look down at something, as this can distort your spinal cord and cause major pain. Make sure that you sleep on your back or on your side, and not on your stomach, as this twists your neck. Walk with your shoulders thrown back rather than hunched over, and avoid leaning inward when sitting down to eat or watch television. If you feel like you have been practicing poor spinal habits and posture for some time, the services of a chiropractor can help readjust your spine and undo the damage.

Muscle tension can be a result and a cause of stress. If your muscles (especially those in the shoulder and neck) are tense, this can cause pain and discomfort, which can lead to bad moods and a general sense of frustration and irritability. Concurrently, an increase in stress (such as that caused by blushing) can in turn cause this muscle tension, which will then increase your stress exponentially! Therefore, it is necessary to stay relaxed and loose at all times possible. To prevent stress, see the section below on meditation and breathing exercises. If you are already tense, then you can buy a massage chair or massage system, employ the services of a professional masseuse, or have a friend give you a massage. The most important areas to focus on are the muscles that lead from your shoulder to the base of your neck. The muscles should feel loose and relaxed. If the muscles are knotty or very firm, then chances are that you could benefit greatly from a massage.

The Power of Meditation and Visualization

We humans just work much better, mentally and physically, when we're relaxed. It's just natural to suffer a loss of performance when we're nervous, stressed, angry, sad, or tense. If you're going to conquer your social anxiety and blushing problems head-on (like you should be doing), then it would be a great boon to be able to stay relaxed and calm during the process to ensure that you are putting your absolute best foot forward. It may seem very difficult to achieve this state of mind under the duress of your issues, and you can't simply tell them to shut up so that you can relax. This is where meditation comes into play.

Meditation may have a bad rap as a spiritual pseudo-prayer activity, and you may be skeptical of its effects. However, meditation is not prayer. It is a physical activity that allows you to clear your mind, which is extraordinarily relaxing and can give your body the boost it needs to meet all of the challenges of the day. There are many different ways to meditate, but it's important to note that meditation is a skill. It takes practice and concentration to achieve consistent results, and it probably won't work well immediately. You need to be persistent.

Below is a great way to begin a meditation routine. After you have mastered these steps, go online and try to expand your meditation though advanced techniques that will increase your relaxation.

1. **Find a silent room, free of visual clutter:** Go to a room in your house or apartment that is reliably silent, with no humming machines or other appliances that generate noise. Also, make sure that the room is clean. Pick the least aggressively-decorated room in the house; the simpler, the better, as elaborate decorations can prompt you to think and can distract you from the process. Sit down on the floor (don't lie down, you don't want to tell your body that you're trying to sleep) and make sure that you are comfortable.

2. **Find a spot on the wall and stare at it:** Find a blank spot on the wall that is noticeable to you. Is there a bump? A difference in the painting strokes? Perhaps a fleck of dirt? Stare at this spot intensely. You will need to do this for a few

minutes to clear your mind of all other thoughts. Whenever you think about something else, just focus on that spot. You can't just try to focus on nothing; your mind will fill with memories or thoughts or worries. You must instead actively try to replace your distracting thoughts with your observations about this single spot on the wall.

3. **Slow your breathing and think about it:** After a few minutes, your brain should be entirely focused on the qualities and characteristics of this spot. You can now begin to breathe deeply, and slow your breathing down. Try to build up to the point where you are taking one long breath every ten seconds. Shift your thoughts from the spot on the wall to the nature of your breathing. Think about how the air feels when it goes into your lungs, the temperature of the air, the speed at which you exhale, or how strongly you blow the air out of your lungs. Continue doing this for twenty to twenty five minutes. Do not close your eyes, or you will feel inclined to go to sleep. After you feel like you have cleared your mind of

all of your thoughts, you may get up and go about your business. You should feel substantially more relaxed.

One Effective Herbal Remedy

If you want to ingest something to help you deal with anxiety but you don't want to take mind-numbing medication, there aren't too many options for you. I have personally spent hundreds of dollars trying various herbal supplements while trying to conquer my own fears, and I had very limited results. However, I did stumble upon something that did help me calm down and reduced my anxiety, especially if I took it before social situations. It is called Passionflower, and it has a calming effect on your body. This was used as a folk remedy in South America for well over five hundred years, and scientists have recently conducted tests to determine if the folk lore had any truth to it. As it turns out, passionflower does have an effect on calming the body, and scientists found it to have similar results to the Benzodiazepine family of drugs, such as Xanax, with fewer side effects. However, you may sometimes experience vomiting or nausea (which I had once or twice), so be careful not to mix it with any other medications, alcohol, or herbal cocktails. This herb is available at health food stores and at herb retailers online, and is usually ingested through adding it to tea or brewing the herb directly (though this option doesn't taste all that great, trust me).

If you effectively combine all of these physical strategies with the mental tricks taught in the previous chapter, then you are well on your way to conquering your anxiety problem and becoming a normal, socially-active person.

If you have implemented the system I have suggested for a period of weeks or months without cheating and have begun to notice results, then read on to the next chapter for hints and tips on how to continue your treatment and recovery.

CHAPTER FIVE

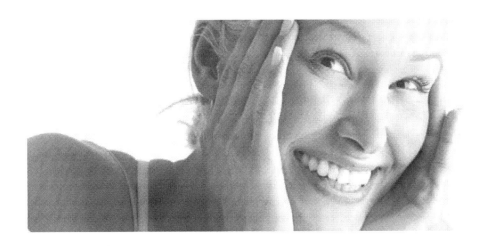

THE NEXT LEVEL

At this point, you've learned the cause of your blushing and what evolutionary functions it plays. You've learned that it's an overreaction and a response to an imaginary problem that you *think* you have. You' learned to practice controlling your mind. You've been making thought logs, and have noted what happens to you when you have an attack. You've even implemented diet, exercise, and meditation into your daily ritual. Congratulations! The hardest part is officially over.

If you've been following all of my instructions for several months and been practicing and implementing my strategies faithfully, then you should have started seeing some progress. You should blush less often, and less intensely. The range of social interactions that you are comfortable with should have grown dramatically, and your fear of these interactions should have fallen sharply.

But....

You don't quite feel all the way better. You feel like there's still something standing in between you and complete normalcy, and you don't know quite how to break through. I know this because I felt the same way. There are several steps I took to further expand my range of comfort and begin to rebuild my social life, and I will share these steps with you. Just a few notes before we begin, though.

One, if you're like me, then there's a good chance that you're pretty hard on yourself. Try to look at your situation objectively and decide if you actually need more work. Because we tend to not be fully aware of how we seem to other people (people with social anxiety are especially bad at this), there's a chance that you've already come further than you think. Also, this may happen to you because you've been giving yourself a hard time for years and years. Your brain may be so used to trying to deal with your problem that it may not recognize that everything's already been fixed! Track your progress by comparing how you felt in the past with how you feel now, or ask a friend or family member if they've noticed any changes. You may be surprised by the answer.

Secondly, the techniques in this chapter are addressed only to people who have completed the previous parts of the Blushing Breakthrough. This manual wasn't designed to be read in a single sitting; rather, it was intended to be digested in parts. If you haven't mastered the techniques described in the first four chapters, then I would hold out on exploring any of these techniques until you have at least started to undo the damage.

If you feel that you're ready, then we can begin. In this chapter, I will cover some material that will help you push yourself over the edge and into a normal life.

Blushing by Location

Why is it, exactly, that we blush in some locations and situations while we remain perfectly calm in others? The answer is simple, and it varies from person to person. Each situation generates what I like to call a Discomfort Rating. This is a score that you assign, from one to ten, to a situation that involves a social interaction. If you still struggle with occasional blushing, it may be related to the specific type of situation that makes you uncomfortable.

Keep a small notepad in your pocket at all times. When you blush or react anxiously to a social situation, write down what that situation was and assign it a Discomfort Rating, with one being the lowest and ten being the highest. Do this for at least several weeks, and then look at your list. You should start to notice similarities between the situations that rate seven or above on your list. Let's talk about why this happens.

It isn't just the presence of people that makes us nervous at this point. We should be relatively comfortable with people in general. It's just that certain situations still make us break out. This could be for several reasons:

- Something about this situation reminds you of a previous anxiety or specific bad experience, and your body pre-empts that experience by sending you a taste of the emotions you felt on that day
- Something about this situation makes you blush because of the circumstantial dynamics (i.e. location, amount of people, type of person,

etc.) represent something you aren't totally comfortable with yet

- Something about the situation is unfamiliar or alien, either emotionally or circumstantially, and you don't fully understand it, so you react nervously and may even have an attack. Below are the top five situations that I struggled with at this stage. I am listing them by their order on the Discomfort Rating scale.

The Top Five Places and Situations that Caused Me to Blush

1. **Nightclubs (Discomfort Rating 9):** This may seem counterintuitive because nobody really notices you in the dark, but for some reason or other, I always felt like a blushing mess in nightclubs and bars long after I had quit blushing everywhere else. This is for several reasons. One, I felt like, in order to successfully be social in a nightclub, you had to try to strike up conversations of interest with members of the opposite sex. Not only did this put pressure and take away the ease of the

social situation, but I also felt that these members of the opposite sex were looking to be impressed, which put additional pressure and tension into the situation.

2. **Walking in to Parties and Social Events (Discomfort Rating 8):** When you first walk into a party, all of the eyes of the rest of the patrons are on you. They give you a quick analysis, and judge you based on your demeanor and physical appearance. I became so uncomfortable with this sensation of being judged that I forgot how to act naturally, and would become a blushing mess for at least five or ten minutes until I felt I had blended in to my surroundings.

3. **Public Speaking (Discomfort Rating 8):** Whenever it was my turn to speak up in public (whether in front of a group of friends, family, church, students, etc.), I always got so nervous because of the sensation that everyone was studying me and waiting for me to please them or entertain them in some way or another.

Needless to say, this made me very nervous, and I usually struggled to remember exactly what it was I had to say.

4. **Introductions (Discomfort Rating 7):** I would get nervous whenever I was introduced to people for several reasons. One, I knew that the first impression was often the most lasting one and the hardest one to undo, so the implied pressure of that social situation caused me to fumble, forget to make eye contact, or to act very curtly. Secondly, introductions tend to involve a lot of small talk. People with social anxiety tend to be pretty bad at small talk because they can't lean back on the topic for shelter or ideas. You have to say something while essentially saying nothing, and act very presentable the entire time. I had a hard time getting people to like me right away because I was so unnerved by the process of meeting people.

5. **Transactions with Clerks (Discomfort Rating 6):** Whenever you order food from a server or request a product from over the counter, you

are making an interaction with a stranger to achieve a specific goal. I would always become tense and uncomfortable if the stranger asked me any questions, or extended the interaction beyond what was strictly necessary. I would come to terms with these situations by rehearsing them in mind, saying "OK, I'm gonna go up to the clerk, ask for some gas, and walk away." If anything didn't go as planned, I would always be very taken aback.

I would now like you to do the same. Look down at your list. What are the top five items on your list? What do they all have in common? Why, exactly, do you feel this way? Which one of the three reasons listed above my list is the source of your discomfort, or is it yet another source? It's crucial that you identify what trains of thought cause you to have a negative reaction. After you have identified these factors, we can apply my formula, which I developed after sitting through hundreds of hours of professional therapy. While the therapy was eventually helpful in that it taught me this method, I can now impart to you this knowledge without needing you to dump your hard-earned money down the tube. You won't need to waste a few hundred hours of time as well, filling a stranger in on your life story in order to help them figure out the source of your problem.

The fact is that recovery is not about analyzing your life story. Recovery is about taking specific actions to eliminate the problem and repeating, repeating, repeating them. Therapists are helpful, but they tend to drag out the discovery phase because it consumes billable time. This is what I came up with.

The Reduction Formula

Look at your top five. What is number five? How uncomfortable do you feel? Do you know exactly why you feel this way? If you do, then you should be able to execute this formula and slowly become more comfortable with this type of situation. This formula has four steps.

1. **Premeditation:** In this step, you really focus in on the "why" of the situation. Why does this circumstance make you feel uncomfortable? Think about the reason repeatedly. We tend to panic and become very afraid of situations we don't understand if we allow our emotions to take us to illogical conclusions. Instead of using your emotions, use your brain and fully understand why you react the way you do to this specific situation. If you gain a strong understanding, you will learn to recognize the cause before it takes effect. This will give you more power over the situation. Your nervous reaction now seems like a logical cause of a specific set of circumstances, which in turns takes a lot of the edge off of the situation and puts you back in control. Plus, the reasons for fearing a situation often seem silly when we are analyzing them within the comfortable confines of our homes, which will go a long way to un-demonize these circumstances.

2. **Observe:** Put yourself in this situation, and take your notebook with you. Lucidly remember or record every single thought you have that leads to a nervous physical reaction or to blushing. Whether this be a memory, a fearful thought, or an illogical observation, write it down and store it away. You will need to make a map of your thought process later. No thought is too irrelevant, so write it all down. You think many things per second, so it may take several tries to get all the information you need.

3. **Analyze:** Once you have gathered enough information about your reaction, build a "train of thought" on a piece of paper that traces the root of your nervous energy from its original thought. Line it up and memorize this train of thought. Then, practice defeating it. You can do this by rehearsing thoughts to interject and interrupt the building thought process. You can simply rehearse it over and over until it loses power over you (because you fear what you do not know the most, this will give you intimate

knowledge of that thought process). You can create smaller-scale situations with less pressure involved and practice re-routing your thoughts and replacing those negative thoughts with confidence. You can have your friends hold a simulation of that circumstance. You can mock the thought process, and use laughter to remove it from a position of power and put you in the driver's seat. I have used combinations of all of these in my own experiences, and each has worked to a different degree depending on the situation.

4. **Apply:** This is, naturally, the most important step in the Reduction Formula. Using your new understanding of your thought process, once again immerse yourself in the situation that makes you uncomfortable. You should be very familiar with what will make you nervous about the situation. When you notice the first thought, apply the disempowering methods to that thought that you practiced within a more comfortable setting. This may not work the first

time or even the second, so it's important to revisit step three with any new observations you have about the circumstance. Eventually, your knowledge of what causes you to become nervous, along with your experience and your thought-slaying technique, will drop that situation a couple points on the Discomfort Rating scale.

This is why I call it the Reduction Formula: every time you execute these for steps, you should be able to expect this circumstance's Discomfort Rating to be reduced by at least one. Once you're comfortable with number five, you can move up to four and continue upwards until you have reduced every situation.

This is similar to what therapists try to do. They make you realize the source of your anxiety, which then robs the anxiety of its power. They then charge you to go practice facing your fear.

But you don't need to pay a therapist to get identical results. Curing anxiety does not come from reflection or analysis, but by *facing your fears head-on and defeating them.* No matter how intelligently the therapist understands your problem, you simply cannot expect to face your fears within the confines of his or her office. This formula combines the analytics of therapy with the practical portion and combines to help you **reprogram your brain.** This is essentially the same thing that Cognitive Behavioral specialists do. They ingrain a new behavior or attitude in your head through repetition until your brain "forgets" how it used to respond!

How to Stop Sweating

Another problem that I had that took quite a while to fix was that whenever I went to meet someone or shake their hand, my own hands were dripping with sweat. Needless to say, this did not help me in my quest to give a good first impression. I used to think that I may have hyperhidrosis, which is the medical term for excessive sweating, but I consulted a doctor, who told me that it was related to my blushing and my social anxiety issues.

If you suffer from excessive sweating and a blushing problem or social anxiety simultaneously, then chances are that the problems are related to one another. Dripping, sweaty palms should be considered a side effect of your condition, not another problem to address. When I began to conquer my social anxiety, I noticed that my sweat condition also disappeared. Being anxious raises our heart rate, which then raises the temperature of your body, which can then cause you to sweat uncontrollably. If you get the anxiety under control via the methods we have discussed, then you shouldn't have to worry about the sweating. However, there are some things you can do to control the sweating.

- **Make sure you're using an antiperspirant as well as a deodorant:** Many people do not look twice at the brand of deodorant that they purchase, immediately assuming that it will help them stop wetness as well as body odor. However, many deodorants function simply as odor killers and do not even attempt to halt the sweating. Ensure that you are purchasing a brand of deodorant that clearly has the word "antiperspirant" printed on the label.

- **Wear cotton:** If you wear artificial fabrics or silk, you are more likely to sweat, because this type of clothing does not allow for the free flow of air and is more likely to cling to your skin when you do begin sweating. Instead, wear cotton, which breathes easily and actually cools the body when you wear it. This will help compensate for the excessive sweating.
- **Wear lighter colors:** If you wear dark colors, your sweat stains will stick out like a giant neon sign. It's very easy to start blushing if you're hyper-aware of your wetness level! Lighter-colored clothes do a good job of disguising the sweating, making you more relaxed and less likely to have incident over the issue.

- **See a doctor:** If recovering from your anxiety doesn't somehow stop the sweating issue, see a doctor. He will be able to tell you if you have hyperhidrosis or not, and will recommend the correct treatment based on that diagnosis.

Small Talk 101

After you've conquered your fear of approaching and conversing with other people, you are going to want to know what to say. Small talk can be an awkward and foreign subject for those who have suffered from social anxiety. We are overwhelmingly afraid of being judged as boring by the other person. The truth is that even the most socially adept people do not have deep, personal conversations with people they have just met. Everyone uses small talk as a way to get a feel for how the person speaks, how they act, and how they carry themselves. Small talk may seem pointless, but we are essentially trying to get a gauge on the other person and decide whether or not we like them when we engage in small talk. Therefore, it is very important to be able to carry out a conversation based around small talk while putting your best foot forward. Here are some basic tips for beginners:

1. **Keep it simple:** It may be tempting to try to talk about your passions in-depth, but this just isn't appropriate for the first meeting. If the other person engages you enthusiastically, then by all means respond. However, the small talk portion of a relationship should avoid taboo topics such as politics and religion (in case you accidentally offend someone) and you should only talk about things that the other person can actively contribute to (nobody likes a lecturer.) The less well you know a person, the simpler the talk needs to be. Talk about the weather, your surroundings, or sports, and see where things lead you. You may be led into a very comfortable conversation just because you were wise enough to keep it simple in the beginning.

2. **Don't try to impress the person:** The key to leaving a good impression through small talk is to be relaxed and natural. If you try too hard to impress them because you feel like you won't stick out from the pack enough, then you are less likely to be successful. People usually distinguish themselves to their friends well after they are already comfortable with them, and the best way to get them comfortable is through small talk. Don't focus on impressing the person or talking excessively about yourself when you meet someone; there will be time for all of that. Make sure you leave a good first impression, and then the rest will fall into place.

3. **Be friendly, but not overly so:** Some people feel vulnerable when they are friendly. However, in reality, other people are just as concerned about what you think of them as much as you are concerned with the opposite. Recognize that you are trying to make the other person feel safe and comfortable by being friendly. Give a firm greeting, listen intently to what the other

person has to say, and react with sympathy or happiness when it is called for. Your kindness will not go unnoticed. It is possible to be too friendly, unfortunately. If you pry too much personal information out of the person, ask too deeply about their personal lives, and stay around much longer than they are wanted, then you run the risk of silencing them for the rest of the night.

4. **Know when to roll off:** The worst possible thing that can happen when you're first meeting someone is the awkward silence that can sometimes squeeze its way into conversations. If you feel like you have been talking to the person to the extent that they have nothing else to say, don't allow an awkward silence to end your conversation. Instead, excuse yourself to use the restroom or to go get another drink or some food. If you leave while you're ahead, you can come back later when you have something to say and still be in the same good standing.

5. **Use confident body language:** People are much more likely to get a good first impression of

someone who is standing up straight, doesn't slouch, uses good manners, firmly shakes hands, and makes eye contact. It is absolutely essential that you pay attention to the signals your body is sending, because they can fly under the radar unless you specifically train yourself to listen and respond.

6. **Tell stories or jokes:** Everyone's got a great story or great joke that's ready for any special occasion. Wait for opportunities to arise naturally in which you can integrate an anecdote or joke into a conversation. You will engage the other party, and hopefully amuse them or make them laugh, which is worth a lot of points in the world of first impressions!

The Four Key Strategies that Public Speakers Employ

Have you ever wondered why brilliant public speakers such as Bill Clinton and Barack Obama are able to stay so calm when you have a miniature freak-out every time you raise your hand or step up to the podium? It's certainly not because they were born with it. Rather, these men have years of practice behind them, and employ the following four tricks to help them stay calm, cool, and collected when making a speech. You can apply the same successful techniques to your own blushing issue, and learn to turn opportunities for public speaking into chances to get valuable practice. I consulted with a Speech coach before I wrote this, and he agreed that there are essentially four major tricks when it comes to staying under control in front of a large group of people.

1. **Ignore the audience:** If you were to recognize exactly how many people you were speaking to, you would become extremely self-aware; it's only natural to freak out when you view the full scope of your audience. With so many people ready to laugh at you if you screw up or trip over your shoes, it's extremely hard to be relaxed. That's why effective public speakers don't even recognize that the audience is there, or they would choke up too! You have to pretend that

the audience is either nonexistent or harmless (pretending they're giant chickens, naked, etc.) We all know that we perform our best when we're natural and calm, and removing the threat of the huge audience goes a long way to helping you feel that way when speaking publicly.

2. **Rehearse:** You may think that you know your speech or presentation front-to-back until you get up to the podium or the front of the room. Then, as if by magic, all of that knowledge evaporates as you realize that you're speaking in front of a group of people, and you look extra-silly as you look like you have nothing to say. Prevent this by rehearsing and re-rehearsing your material. Do it in formal settings, like in front of friends or family members, in order to practice having a listener. Make reference points throughout your presentation or speech that you can use to find yourself in case you get distracted by your audience and become lost.

3. **Have Confidence:** Many people are paralyzed of public speaking; you don't need to have a blushing issue in order to have this fear. Unfortunately, for people like us, our fear and emotional backlash is extra-intense. If you approach the situation full of dread, thinking that you will freak out, then you most certainly will. Use your positive feedback loops (covered in Chapter Three) to build some interior confidence before stepping out on stage. If you believe in yourself and your abilities, then you are much more likely to get through the speech.

4. **Take your time:** Time seems to pass at half of its normal rate when you're up in front of a large group of people, so it's easy to lose track of how fast you're talking. Most people rush incoherently through the speeches, leaving audience members confused and befuddled. This can be because the speaker wants to get the process over with, or because he or she is nervous and not aware of the pace at which they are talking. Do yourself a favor and force

yourself to slow down. Write "Slow Down" periodically on your index cards or speech notes so that you can maintain a lucid and clear pattern of speech throughout the presentation.

In this chapter, I've broken down some of the solutions to the problems I encountered well into my own recovery process. If you continue to expand your horizons, challenge yourself socially, and never become complacent, then you will realize one happy day that your social anxiety and blushing problems are a thing of the past.

AFTERWORD

Do you remember my story from the opening moments of this book? Do you remember how crippled I was, how paralyzed by even the thought of a social situation occurring? Did you feel the same way?

Millions of people all over the globe suffer from excessive blushing and social anxiety disorder just like you and I did. It can be an intimidating problem. You can be led to feel like an outcast, or like something is wrong with you. You can feel like you will never, ever get better.

Wrong! As you now know, social anxiety was a small hill rather than an insurmountable mountain chain. The techniques in this manual have taught you how to understand your condition and how to attack it. You may not be one hundred percent cured, but this will come naturally in time, as you have undone the mental mistakes and reprogrammed your mind to think in more productive channels.

Never, ever stop trying to improve yourself! Keep conquering social barriers and making new friends until you achieve what you thought was a pipe-dream of a goal: **HAPPINESS.** When you reap the rewards of your personal hard work and of attacking your problems directly, you will experience feelings of contentment and satisfaction that you thought were previously out of your reach. How do I know this? *Because it happened to me!* It didn't happen overnight; I had to work on developing my system and tweaking the finer points through embarrassing trial and error. But, deep inside, I knew that if I tried hard enough and was persistent enough, I would make it through my trials intact and become a stronger person because of them. If you follow in my footsteps, then you can too.

Let's revisit the list of the nine emotions that cause blushing and review how you've defeated them or how you've prepared yourself for them.

1. **Shame:** Once you've conquered your anxiety, you learn to recognize that everyone in the world makes embarrassing mistakes. It's only human. You should never be overly hard on yourself; try laughing it off instead! People will relate to you rather than laugh at you.

2. **Humiliation:** Your new confidence and swagger are untouchable by the mere thoughts and comments of a single individual. You've learned by now that you can't please everyone. If someone is humiliating you, you shouldn't feel embarrassed. Just walk away and talk to someone who respects you for who you are.

3. **Shyness:** Because you've practiced techniques for meeting new people and staying calm and relaxed during social situations, you're no longer afraid to speak your mind or introduce yourself to someone. Kiss those red faces, sweaty palms, and awkward looks goodbye.

4. **Gratitude:** If you've followed all of the instructions in this book, you will recognize that helping each other out is a natural part of human relations. You should be able to tactfully thank someone without feeling your face turn red.

5. **Love or Intense Emotionality:** Because you've learned that you deserve these affections through your positive feedback loops and daily morning notes, you should no longer be humbled or overwhelmed when this occurs. Enjoy it!

6. **Recognition:** Because you've learned to stay calm when all eyes are on you, you should be able to accept praise and recognition graciously and confidently, not turn into a tomato.

7. **Exposure:** You have learned to keep your cool in public places and to relax when the spotlight is on you. This will never feel entirely comfortable, but you should be able to be aware of your bodily reactions and keep them under control.

8. **Pressure:** Because you've learned meditation, physical exercises, and mental tricks to keep yourself focused on your goals, pressure should be a welcome opportunity to prove yourself rather than a demonic specter that ruins your day.

9. **Anticipation:** Because you have destroyed your perception that social situations are harmful, you should now look forward to parties and events rather than fear them.

If this is how you feel when confronted with these nine emotions, then CONGRATULATIONS!!!

You've come a long way. It's been a rough journey, but nothing ever worth doing is easy.

So go out and enjoy the world! You'll benefit from your new knowledge that the Earth is full of people who share your interest, beliefs, and goals. All you have to do is find them!

Made in the USA
Lexington, KY
03 November 2010